I0141107

Living Authentically

WITH LIFE'S CHALLENGES AND UNCERTAINTY

Sylvia Fortnam

Cover image courtesy of Gerd Altmann

Special thanks to Jessica Rose Photography

MELBOURNE AUSTRALIA

Sylvia Fortnam c/- Intertype
Unit 45, 125 Highbury Road
BURWOOD VIC 3125
www.intertype.com.au

Book Layout ©2019 Intertype
Cover Image Courtesy of Gerd Altmann
Special thanks to Jessica Rose Photography

Ordering Information:
Quantity sales. Special discounts are available on quantity purchases by cor-
porations, associations, and others. For details, contact the "Special Sales
Department" at the address above.

Living Authentically / Sylvia Fortnam —1st ed.
ISBN 978-0-6485960-9-7

Book Reviews

Sylvia should be congratulated on providing a heartfelt and honest portrayal of her experiences dealing with recurring metastatic cancer. I am moved and touched by her personal story and journey, as you will be too. The courage and stamina she has displayed is remarkable. Sylvia has defied all odds through her own deep honest inner work, guided by the help of her doctors, health practitioners and many friends, loved ones, family and support people. She has done so remarkably well. When you look at Sylvia she radiates love, strength, energy, humour and vibrant health despite what her tests may show. She is a great role model for many patients who are experiencing a life threatening illness - *A/Professor Vicki Kotsirilos AM, MBBS, FACNEM, FASLM, Awarded Honorary Fellowship of the RACGP*

This book is a poignant, enlightening and uplifting account of what is an intensely personal journey of a woman and her people dealing with the ongoing diagnosis of cancer. Reading it has given me an insight into how someone manages to still keep on going whilst living, loving and growing authentically despite the devastating hand they have been dealt. I hope this book shows the reader that a challenging diagnosis doesn't need to define or dictate how you live your life. That when you're ready and you feel your moment of willingness and courage is here, you discover that you do have choice in how you want to live - *Joanne O'Sullivan Oncology Nurse*

Sylvia shows us that it is possible to live compassionately and authentically through the most difficult times. And that like Sylvia, at some point in our life we have all lived with uncertainty and loss. When I first met Sylvia she sought permanent freedom from fear. What she showed throughout our sessions was a capacity to be open, vulnerable and fragile while she lovingly observed and sat with her fears. Her capacity to do this, with much love and self compassion, allowed her to be fully present to herself and more able to know and tend to whatever she emotionally needed at the time. Sylvia I admire your courageous spirit. Thank you for the gift you have given in writing this book. It teaches us, as your title suggests, that it is possible to live an authentic life 'with' life's challenges and uncertainties - *Vicki Holmes Psychologist*

Reading Sylvia's book was very insightful for me. It helped me to really understand the emotional journey of what people go through whilst living with cancer. I was blown away by her courage and determination to face her fears, disappointments and grief so authentically. The healing her family has gone through with her on this journey was so heart warming. Through every page I felt Sylvia's beautiful heart. Her message in this book is needed . I have passed copies on to others in the hope that it helps them with their own personal cancer journey. Sylvia is such a light of hope, inspiration and love - *Angela D'Amelio Yoga Teacher, Holistic Counsellor, Reiki Practitioner and Teacher*

Contents

Dedication

My beautiful family David, Chris, Di and Brendon
Sarah, Beecher and Jess
Indi, Harper, Addison, Evie, Jimmy, Wilder and Reef
My awesome family, friends, medical/complementary and
spiritual team

All my love always

Ovarian Cancer Research Foundation

Proceeds from the sale of this book help further the valuable work of the Ovarian Cancer Research Foundation.

Established in 2000, the Ovarian Cancer Research Foundation (OCRF) has grown to become Australia's leading independent body dedicated to funding national ovarian cancer research.

They demonstrate leadership in the ovarian cancer space through:
- Prioritising research that will have the biggest impact for the most women
- Collaborating with ovarian cancer experts to identify and pursue the most promising projects
- Embracing a dual focus on both the present (reducing the lethal threat for women today) and the future (striving for complete eradication of ovarian cancer)

www.ocrf.com.au

Forward

I was diagnosed with an aggressive breast cancer in 1999 and went into remission after six months of treatment. I have never had breast cancer since.

In 2011 I was diagnosed with a Grade 3c Ovarian Cancer which had metastasised throughout my abdomen. In 2012 I was diagnosed with the BRCA 1 Gene mutation.

This book is my emotional journey with cancer since that 2011 diagnosis and my being able to finally live authentically with the uncertainty of an ongoing life-threatening disease.

I feel blessed to be sharing my life with my husband of forty-two years, my three adult children, their partners, and our seven beautiful grandchildren.

My family and friends are the joy and love in my life.

All that I meet and all that have shared my life's journey with me have been my greatest teachers in helping me to open my heart and mind more deeply to what life is calling for in each moment.

I am so grateful to have had the opportunity to live a more compassionate, loving life, staying true to what resonates deeply within me.

With love
Sylv

Preface

When I was first diagnosed with ovarian cancer in 2011 I was terrified. As my journey unfolded I discovered that I have choice in my living and dying authentically.

Having been diagnosed with cancer 6 times with the medical opinion that if I don't get hit by a bus, have a car accident, suffer a heart attack or die from any other number of causes of death, cancer will probably be what brings death to this body.

I have felt my sadness and grief in knowing my body will die one day. And I've grieved more deeply watching my family's grief and fears.

Cancer has shown me that if I'm willing to stay open to what's presenting in my life in the present moment, without adding my story or getting lost in my thoughts, there's a beautiful quiet clarity present, and my fears don't 'stick' to anything. They still arise, but they don't stay for long because I'm not feeding them or adding to them. I can acknowledge fear is here, sit with it, feel it, and watch the fear pass – most of the time.

My feelings of sadness and grief take longer to pass though, as in my heart I want to be with my family and friends, both physically and mentally, for as long as I can. I'm aware that I'm more attached to my thoughts and stories when grief and sadness are present, and I'm ok with that too in the end, because I also recognise that's it's the love I feel for them all that drives that wanting to stay.

In January this year I rang my Oncologist in tears because I sensed that the chemo wasn't working and I stepped into "OMG this is IT!!"

I didn't like the unsettled, uncertain, scared space I was in, but that passed when I gave myself the time to sit with the fear and allow it to just be fear and nothing else, because I really didn't know if that was the final "IT".

I have had days where I've felt totally lost in my sadness and fears. Days where I'd reached the point of feeling so tired with the uncertainty and unknown of this journey that it became overwhelming for me and I withdrew from the world and wished with all of my heart that cancer wasn't in my life.

But at the moment it is. So, what do I do? How do I live with this?

Having also felt and lived great joy, love and gratitude in the midst of cancer, I've discovered that I do have a choice in how I want to be, and that all the emotions I feel; fear, hope, sadness, grief, hopelessness, disappointment, love, celebration, they're all ok and part of living an honest, rich and full life.

I have been given the opportunity to live every day knowing that death will definitely come to this body which has morphed into my mantra of: "Ok, then how do I want to live?"

The irony for me is, yes, I choose to focus on life and living, acknowledging the love, joy and gratitude that's so present for me every day whilst also knowing that death is a given.

Life is here to be lived as its calling to be lived. Death will take care of itself. I don't know how or when death will come, so I choose to focus on Life.

As my journey continues to unfold, I don't know what will happen next, but I do know that I'm choosing to live from the honesty and authenticity of what's wanting to be felt, expressed and lived. Whenever I ask myself, "Well, I'm still here, so how do I want to live?"

My answer is this: I want to open myself fully to the life and love that I'm so blessed to be a part of, and from that space let's see what today brings.

I want to help bring some relief around the fear of death, and to shine a light on the fact that we have no control over our body dying one day, but we do have control over how we choose to live.

Seeing and living the beauty and honesty in Life, and seeing the beauty and peace that Death can be, feels very comforting to me and is a choice that I'm happy to live from.

There are people actively dying that teach us that death can be a beautiful process, a true returning to home, to love; and to those people I am truly grateful.

With much love

Sylv x

Addendum : July 2019

At the time of completing this book I thought I was cancer free, however in November 2018 a PET scan showed that cancer had returned. I started chemo in December 2018 but this time the treatment didn't work and I'm not in remission yet. There are also no trials I can access at the moment. The only option for me so far is to try a different chemo. If that doesn't work I'm not sure what will come next. I've chosen to delay further treatment for a while to give my body time to heal.

I'm still choosing to live a healthy, loving lifestyle, and continue to have my complementary therapies. I'm not feeling any fear at the moment about dying, but I do feel sadness and grief at times as I watch my family go through their grief and sadness with this latest news. And, as much as I 'know' to live in the now, there are still times I step into the future and feel the sadness of missing them all when I physically die.

If I compare all the roller coaster emotions that come up for me, happiness, fun, laughter and the loving connections I'm so blessed to have far outweigh the moments of sadness and grief.

My life is beautiful

CHAPTER 1

Terror and Beauty - 2011

When I was told that I had Grade 3c Ovarian cancer in 2011 I was terrified. I was convinced I'd be dead within six weeks.

I was moving between sobbing my heart out and going completely numb. David and I would hug each other and just cry. We tried to distract ourselves by going to the movies or watching DVD's, but at the end of the movie we'd just cry. We tried really hard not to, because we wanted to be strong for each other, but we couldn't do it. So we just surrendered to how scared and sad we were and cried.

We'd lie in bed at night looking up at our bedroom ceiling which was covered with fluorescent stars and planets glowing in the dark, and talk about what we thought happens to you when you die.

Those nights were the most heart opening, honest, soul connecting nights we'd ever felt in all the years we've been together. We bonded on such a deep level. It was beautiful.

That was the gift in that diagnosis. The deeper love and connection we felt for each other.

The scary bit was knowing that the life I'd known was forever gone, and the belief that I was going to die very soon.

There'd be days when I'd be driving in my car seeing people go about their daily business thinking how lucky they were not to have to worry about dying.

I remember driving to the supermarket one night with David and watching a man putting his rubbish bins out. "He's going to die one day too" popped into my head, and somehow that thought helped me to feel less alone.

FACT: *Millions of people have died before me and millions will die after me.*

I had surgery to remove as much of the cancer as possible and then had six months of chemo.

The great news was I went into remission very quickly, and I coped really well with the whole regime.

The oncology nurses were amazing. Full of great humour and deep caring. They have the patience of saints and were brilliant at reading my emotions and helping me with any concerns or fears I may have been feeling.

My oncologist Gary, was awesome. His confidence and expertise gave me confidence, and the fact that I was responding so well to the treatment helped my spirits rise.

David and I always came out of Gary's office feeling great. There was always a lot of laughter in those rooms.

I would tend to bombard Gary with loads of questions every time I saw him. Sometimes asking was great, sometimes it wasn't so great as I didn't always like the honest answers I got. Sometimes I'd think "You know what? Just lie to me. Let me have some peace of mind on this one."

But the logical, survival part of me knew I had to know the truth. What I found particularly hard to cope with was the waiting for my test results, and the "we don't know" answers. "Everyone's different. Everybody responds differently."

I wanted assurances.

Part of this cancer stuff is a journey of data collecting through trials, stats and percentages, so there's an average outcome, but there's no guarantees. And I wanted guarantees. I like my safety nets, I like to know that: "Yes Sylv, 100% this will definitely work and you'll be cured forever."

But nobody can give me that.

Life's not like that.

I became stricter with what I ate and drank, used complementary therapies, always running it by Gary first, was spiritually supported by a loving, caring Tibetan Buddhist community, and I was surrounded by family and friends who genuinely loved and cared about me. I felt very grateful to be so beautifully blessed in what started as a scary journey for me.

By the end of my treatment I felt wonderful! Optimistic and completely confident that I was going to live a cancer free life. After all, I'd gone into remission early and the data showed that most women who responded as well as I had to treatment had a good chance of being cured provided the cancer didn't return within a four-year period.

In my mind that was easily achievable

CHAPTER 2

Cancer Free - 2012

In 2012 my surgeon suggested I be tested for the BRCA 1 gene mutation as I'd had an aggressive breast cancer when I was 41 (in 1999) and to then get ovarian cancer at 53 brought up a red flag for him.

There's not a lot of history of breast cancer in my family. Only a great aunt on my dad's side who died at 54. Because of this I would never have been eligible for the free genetic testing prior to the ovarian cancer diagnosis. And because my dad comes from a family of all boys the likelihood of any breast cancer history was minimised.

So I had a choice to make.

Do I take the test and know for sure and help other family members to work with the information that's discovered? Or do I not be tested and just continue on, don't rock the boat? Ignorance is bliss - right?

I had a daughter and a grand-daughter, the choice was easy for me.

After the gene mutation had been confirmed, I was asked if my parents would be open to being tested. They were, and the results showed my dad was the carrier. That was really hard for him as he stepped into guilt. He blamed himself. I remember him saying to me "I'm so sorry kid. I gave this to you." My heart felt so sad for him. I hugged him and said: "Dad, it's not your fault. You didn't purposely give this to me."

He agreed but I could still see the sadness in his eyes.

I'll be honest, there have been one or two times that I wished I didn't know. That I didn't have to carry that knowledge around in my head. But ensuring that those I love are informed and can prevent having a similar journey to mine is really important to me.

In the end you do find ways of living with what life brings you. As one of my gorgeous girlfriends once said to me:

"It's like having white noise going on in the back of your mind. You're not consciously living from it, but you know it's always there."

The blessing of my being tested is how far reaching this has been for every person in both my immediate and extended family. They can all be tested for free and put preventative measures into place now if they want to.

When I was first told I had this genetic condition I wanted to cry. I felt that any control I had over this cancer had been ripped out of my arms. Up until being given this news I was very confident that all would be well. I'd been so sure I wasn't a carrier. After all, I had breast cancer over twelve years ago and that never came back. How could I have a BRCA 1 gene mutation?

The solid ground I'd been standing on was beginning to crack. My confidence was shaky. I felt like I was losing my safety net.

My breast specialist wanted me to consider a double mastectomy after she'd been informed of my genetic testing. I was horrified at the thought initially. I understood that she wanted to give me the best possible outcome for living a long cancer free life, but somehow for me it felt like such a drastic thing to do when I'd been breast cancer free for so long.

I looked at the websites she'd suggested and read the comments of many women who'd had this surgery, and after a while I felt, well, if it's going to give me better odds I'll do it.

I was also told that having this operation was only an option if the ovarian cancer didn't come back, and as I was cancer free so far it seemed the right time to look into it.

I still needed my safety net. Something I could fall back on to help me feel more stable in my life. To help keep the fear of cancer at bay.

CHAPTER 3

Devastated and Humbled – Early 2013

"Your tumour markers have gone up slightly."

"Ok. So what do we do now?"

"We wait and see what happens. If they continue to go up we'll do some tests."

I had a mini melt down. Not in Gary's rooms. At home. I could feel the fear creeping back. That feeling of uncomfortableness. Uncertainty. And all of these feelings morphed into an absolute knowing that I was terrified of the unknown. I hated having to wait and see what my tumour markers were doing.

I couldn't be tested too early because the scans won't detect any cancer if it's too small. So you have to wait.

Again I'm oscillating between: "I feel so good it can't be cancer" to:

"Nooooo I don't want cancer to be back!!"

I'd lie in bed searching my body for any lumps or sore spots, feeling relieved if I couldn't find any and reassuring myself that all was well.

And then on another day I'd feel some pain and be reminded of what the cancer felt like the last time I had it. "It must be back" is where I'd mentally go in those moments. I became hyper vigilant. The mental strain of constantly scanning my body and listening to the talk in my head going to and fro was exhausting and yet I couldn't sleep.

August 2013

Finally my markers were high enough to warrant testing.

I remember waking up the morning I was to see Gary to get my test results. It was a beautiful sunny day. I was so sure everything was going to be ok. I'd found some peace and comfort in thinking: "Well if it's back I'll just have chemo again, go into remission, and then I'll be cancer free for the rest of my life."

I felt this was a really doable outcome for me.

So into Gary's rooms I went. He doesn't look his usual cheery self, but I don't connect that with my results. He also has a trainee oncologist present.

Introductions are made and I ask:

"So what are the results?"

"It's back."

I can't remember Gary's exact words or in what order things came out, but the gist of it was this:

In most cases, if ovarian cancer comes back within a four year period, it's probably going to keep coming back. I felt deflated. Devastated. I do remember saying something like:

"I hope you don't mind me swearing", not waiting for an answer, and a long, drawn out, "Fuuuuuccckkkk" popping out. Followed by a few more shorter versions, because I just couldn't believe what I'd heard. My brain wouldn't compute properly. That's not what I had planned.

No one battered an eye at my reaction.

I'd asked David not to ask how long I've got if the cancer was back, which he honoured. But for some reason that I couldn't explain at the time that question blurted out of my mouth. To which Gary did give me an estimated time. But as we all know, no one really knows because every body and mind is uniquely different. And a part of me was relieved to know "Well at least I've got more than six months to live!" And another part of me went into fear because I was being told I was going to die one day.

My safety net was tattered

I sat with "Why the hell did I ask that?"

And the beautiful answer I got was:

Because I needed to know I had more than six months to live.

Because I wasn't ready to die.

Because I want to be here for as long as I can.

And I was at peace with that answer.

I'd never really experienced the serious side of Gary before, so I said to David that at my next appointment I was going to ask him to relate to me in a certain way. I was worried that all my visits were going to become heavy and serious and I didn't want that, so before I went to have my first chemo treatment this is what I asked for:

When I come into your office I don't want to see "Dead woman walking" in your eyes.

I still want you to high five me every time my tumour markers have dropped; and

I want you to give me a gold star when I go into remission.

He gave me 2

On my first appointment with Gary after being told the cancer was back I walked into his rooms loaded up with questions and photocopies of different treatments that were available or being tried. He sat there reading through everything I'd brought in. He made a few piles.

"No."

"Not enough evidence."

"You can try that treatment if you want to but it hasn't had a high success rate" (to which I thought - nope I want to go with what's worked with a high success rate).

"We used to do that, but it was too damaging to the body."

"That treatment isn't for ovarian cancer."

He also looked up half way through reading that pile and said, "Geez you could have drip fed me these!!"

To which David and I just cracked up laughing. That's the magic of Gary. We could all still laugh. He helped lighten that journey for us. (He still does!!)

I think it was on my second or third visit to Gary that I said:

"I can't do this by myself, I need help."

I felt so devastated that the cancer had returned. The peace I'd found believing I'd get a second chance to live a cancer free life when I went into remission was shattered.

Again I cried a lot. David and I would go to meet my sister and brother-in-law at a cafe and he'd have to ring them and cancel because I'd be sitting there crying, feeling embarrassed, and wanting to go home. I couldn't go out. I was constantly thinking about my death. I'd try to remember to live. To focus on the beauty and love that was in my life, but then I'd cry more because I was already missing them in my mind. And I was sad because I knew that this wasn't just impacting me. It was affecting the people I loved. I felt I was the source of their unhappiness and fears, that I was a burden to them.

At times I wanted to run away and not tell anyone where I was, hoping that my not being in their lives would spare them any further sorrow. I used to say to David:

"I'm so sorry you have to go through this."

To which he'd always say:

"I love you. I don't want to be anywhere else, we'll get through this together."

I did confess to David that at times I felt it would be easier for him if I just left. His answer to that was it would be harder for him. He wanted me to be in his life. To share in his life.

That was the beauty of this second diagnosis.

The depth of David's love and commitment was so humbling to me.

Gary referred me to an Oncology Psychologist named Jane who was brilliant in really challenging me in the way I was thinking.

She helped me to see that I was still looking to other people to validate myself. She helped me to see how I was ever so subtly still saying:

"Here's my life tell me how to live it."

She helped me to live and stand strong in what my truth was, what resonated for me in my life.

And I remember sitting in her office one day, feeling really stuck in the sadness of missing everyone when I die, to which Jane said:

"Sylv, you're not dead yet!!"

And other gems like:

"You know it might not be cancer that kills you, you could get hit by a bus." (Weirdly I got comfort from that, cause there's a part of me that just doesn't want to die from cancer).

"What's your truth? Not what you've read or accepted from someone else. What's *your* truth?"

"Everyone's going to die one day, you've just got more information than most people."

"You don't know when you're going to die. Even on your death bed you don't know when your last breath will be."

"Nobody really knows what happens when you die."

"Embrace the unknown" ("Yeah right!" is what instantly went through my mind. I wasn't quite ready for that one).

"Be curious about whatever comes up. Watch it with curiosity."

"Look at your fear with curiosity."

(I really struggled with that because I actually became my fear whenever it came up. My whole body would shake sometimes and I'd feel lost. I actually thought I was having a heart attack one night. The pain in my chest was acute and it hurt to breathe. I sat up partially in bed and started consciously focusing on breathing deeply. I timed myself and promised if the pain was still there by a certain time I'd ring an ambulance. But because I could feel it easing every time I relaxed a little, there was a part of me that eventually knew it probably wasn't my heart. It lasted half an hour. My GP said it was an anxiety attack).

"You're not you're fear."

(That was a real light bulb moment for me. Stopped me in my tracks. I'd heard and read this statement many times but never really got it. This time I did).

Jane put me onto some great books, meditation cds and quoted Leunig, an Australian artist, poet, philosopher and cartoonist.

She helped me live, not just conceptualise, about living in the now, because:

FACT: *That's all we really have. The past is gone and the future hasn't happened yet.*

She quoted a passage from a book written by a woman who was living with a life-threatening illness. I can't remember it exactly, but this is how I interpreted it.

You're skating in the middle of a frozen lake when the ice starts to crack. You know you can't make it back to the bank and that you're going to fall in and die. What do you do?

I think the author was saying:

I can't do anything about this but I can choose how I'm going to live my last few moments before I die.

So the logical part of my mind thinks:

"Oh, the right answer for this is me sitting down calmly and choosing to live these moments gracefully because I can't change or control the outcome of dying. Death is a given. How do you want to live your final moments?"

But the truth for me, the image I had, was me on all fours crawling as slowly, lightly and carefully as I could, hoping I'd make it to the banks before the ice cracked all the way through.

I don't think I gave Jane the right answer, but I gave her what was the truth for me in that moment.

Through my sessions with Jane I was inspired to write a little piece called "Searching for Peace" which I'll add to the end of this book.

Writing this helped give me some clarity about how I really felt about certain beliefs I'd been holding and why I was so desperate to feel at peace when it came time for me to die.

So far this cancer journey was blowing my complacency about life and some strongly held beliefs out of the water.

My safety net was tattered.

I didn't breeze through the chemo regime as smoothly this time. I was on a different chemo combination. It'd take me a couple of days to bounce back, and that added to my fear.

I noticed that every time I felt exhausted or unwell it triggered the fear of death for me. Like a chain reaction, everything that felt negative in my life would pop up. I'd sit with these feelings and really look at them. It felt like once the trigger was activated wave after wave of negativity would show itself and the overwhelming emotion was the fear of me dying, followed by the sadness of missing my family and friends, because at this stage I had come to realise that :

FACT: *I'm going to die one day and there's nothing I can do to stop that. It's a given. That's the cycle every living thing on this planet follows. No escaping it. You're born, you have a life for however long, then you die.*

Ironically, sometimes when I really surrendered to the truth of this, I'd feel peaceful and this question would always come up:

"Ok, if I have no control over death. If I'm fully accepting that death is a given:

HOW DO I WANT TO LIVE?"

And when I flowed from the core of that question, without editing it, without analysing it, this is what spontaneously came out:

I want to live from the loving space of an open heart.

I want to acknowledge and live the happiness that's present in my life.

I want to live authentically.

I want to live from the heart of a truth that's rooted in kindness and courage.

I want to live in this present moment knowing that I am Life itself.

Because I noticed that when I could allow myself to stay in the now, when I wasn't following and believing the thoughts and stories in my head, my life was pretty awesome. I was surrounded by family and friends who had the courage and love to walk beside me. Who didn't see a victim of cancer standing in front of them. Who could genuinely laugh with me and focus on all that was good in our lives. Who gave me the space to sit with my sadness and fears, to really listen to me.

One sister (my "cafe buddy" and best friend) in particular is brilliant at this. She'll allow me my space, but she won't let me wallow. She'd always text or ring me and sometimes she'd just come over if she felt I was distancing myself for too long.

The love, support and prayers of my beautiful spiritual friends, Lama Tendar (a very compassionate Tibetan Buddhist monk) and his Sangha, also gave me great comfort.

How blessed am I!!

So blessed.

I can still love, laugh, cry, walk, talk (too much sometimes!!), experience life, pray, dance, have fun, travel, shop, have lunch with my beautiful friends (I love food!!). The list is long.

Cancer doesn't define me. It's not me, not the true me.

Gary was confident I'd go into remission again. And true to his word I did.

CHAPTER 4

Remission – November 2013 to August 2014

From my 2013 diagnosis I decided to live an even "cleaner" life to ensure I'd be cancer free. I found room to improve on my previous lifestyle. I was mentally supported by a great psychologist, and beautiful family and friends. Physically I had a great medical team in my oncologist, oncology nurses and GP. Spiritually I had the support and prayers of loving friends, a beautiful Tibetan Buddhist community and a brilliant kinesiologist. I'd also have occasional energy healings. I found great comfort in the teachings of Jesus, Buddha, Gangaji and Adyashanti, and I loved reading the Dalai Lamas' books and going to see him whenever he was in Melbourne.

My weight dropped significantly and I remember asking Gary once: "Why am I so yellow?" I was concerned my liver wasn't coping with my past treatments.

Turned out it was all the carrots I'd been eating!! They were my "go to" snack in between meals.

I remember having dinner with my brother and sister-in-law in a little country pub one night. She commented on how strict I was in regards to my food. I shared with her that I wanted to give myself the best possible chance of living a cancer free life.

What I discovered about myself during 2013/2014 was how hard fear was driving every bit of nourishment I was putting into my body. How fast I was running trying to avoid cancer. Trying to spare myself the terror of reliving yet another cancer diagnosis. I wasn't living in the now, I was living in the future, trying to prevent cancer from happening. Food was my way of feeling I had some control over it. But I wasn't fully enjoying it. I was always scanning to make sure I was eating the "right" food.

Some of the unhelpful things I said to myself during this time were:

I've done something to bring the cancer back.
Hadn't done enough to prevent it.
Should have had more juices.
Not had that fear or thought - that's why it came back.
I wasn't mentally positive enough.

Self judgement
Self blame
Guilt

My sister was worried that I was getting too thin, but I was determined to heal myself of this cancer. I wasn't going to give it any opportunities to grow back.

But grow back it did.

CHAPTER 5

Disappointment, Reflection and Trust – 2014

W hen cancer returned in August 2014 I was scared and disappointed. But surprisingly not terrified.

A feeling of: "Well, this is it then. I'm going to die from this" filled me.

I had loving and deep conversations with my husband, children, family members and friends about death and my wish to not leave this earth with any regrets.

I hoped I would die knowing I'd helped at least one person in a positive way. That I wasn't leaving this life feeling unfinished. And that when it came time for me to die, I'd be at peace with it. That death wouldn't be the scary monster I'd imagined it to be.

Being at peace with my death was a driving force for me since my first diagnosis in 2011. It was really important to me. Whenever I sat with Why? the truth was because if I'm at peace with death I won't be afraid of dying. Peace is a much nicer feeling than fear is. I also real-ised that my body instinctively knows how to die. There's a process to it, a wisdom, and if I could trust that I'd be ok. But my mind and sur-vival instincts are strong so I didn't stay in that body wisdom for very long, which on reflection is sad because I did feel a beautiful quietness come over me when I really sat with that wisdom, that knowing.

Synchronicity and Trust

When I was diagnosed with cancer in 2014 my eldest son, Chris, (who along with his dad, my David, was always looking up new trials on the internet for me) rang me to let me know a trial was starting for women with Recurrent Ovarian Cancer. I looked up the website and sent an email saying I was keen to participate in this.

From there I spoke to Oncologist Assoc/Professor Linda Mileshkin who worked from both The Mercy Hospital For Women in Heidelberg and Peter Mac. She helped me understand the process and criteria I needed to follow to get onto the trial.

Gary, my oncologist, was on board immediately and did everything he could to ensure I met this criteria.

The trial was called Solo 2.

I was driving home from Cabrini Hospital one afternoon with David when I got a phone call from Gary's receptionist telling me I had an appointment for an interview at The Mercy Hospital. As we were speaking a four-wheel drive BMW overtook us with the number plate SOLO 2.

I was slapping David's arm and pointing to the car in amazement and this beautiful sense of "OMG!! I'm going to get onto this trial!" came over me. What are the odds that as I'm being told I have an appointment for this trial that a car with that particular number plate pulls up in front of us?

Some would say Coincidence.

My heart said Sign.

There were a few hairy moments when I thought I wasn't going to make it and I'd feel shaky and scared. But then I'd remember that number plate and the circumstances in which I saw it and how I felt seeing it. I decided I was going to trust that feeling.

I received a phone call from The Mercy about three quarters of the way through my chemo treatments from a staff member who told me that there was no guarantee I was a definite for this trial. That was contrary to what my oncologist had told me. So I rang Gary and he reassured me that I was definitely meeting all the necessary criteria and would be eligible for Solo 2.

Once my chemo treatments were all finished and I was in remission again, Gary wished me well as I was now going to be referred to Assoc/Professor Linda Mileshkin who was in charge of the Solo 2 project. I hadn't really thought about that and felt a bit sad at leaving Gary's care. I remember asking him that day if I had to have all the blood tests and scans that had to be taken during the trial period, to which he just eyeballed me and said:

"You want the trial - you do the tests."

Fair enough.

I received a phone call not long after this from Linda to say that they had enough people so I wouldn't be needed.

My heart sank.

But then she went on to say that I was able to be a part of what they called The Access Programme.

This meant I would actually get the drug Olaparib (and not have to be subjected to the protocol of a certain percentage of trial people receiving a placebo). It also meant I didn't have to have any scans, AND I was able to continue seeing Gary as my oncologist!! How blessed was I!!

I felt so grateful for what I'd received I started to cry and thanked Linda for all her help and kindness in my Solo 2 journey.

CHAPTER 6

Starting The Trial Drug Olaparib - 2015

I started taking Olaparib on the 7th January 2015, two days before my 57th birthday.

Gary told me I needed to have blood tests and appointments every four weeks to ensure my body was coping with the new drug. Once it was clear all was well it moved to every six weeks which also coincided with six weekly port flushes. (I had a port put in in 2013 for my chemo treatments as the veins in my arm aren't great).

David took a photo of me holding my first tablet and we joked how the white capsules with black stripes were a good omen because they were the colour of his beloved footy team Collingwood.

We were filled with hope and I felt I could breathe again. Like I'd been given a reprieve. David and I went away for a weekend to Williamstown with light hearts and much happiness.

My safety net was well and truly back and I was keen to dive back into life.

For the rest of this year I happily did on line courses, mainly with Adyashanti, listened to radio broadcasts of Gangaji and started seeing clients again.

Although for most of 2015 I felt very fulfilled, humbled and at peace, I noticed that if my safety net felt threatened, the fear of cancer returning would still arise and I'd feel disappointed that it was still there.

There were times when I couldn't get my Olaparib tablets because they were coming to Australia from the UK and for reasons like postal strikes or shipping delays I might have to go a few days or a week without them.

The protocol was, Gary would write a one month prescription for me and I'd take that prescription down to the Cabrini Hospital pharmacy. We were only allowed one month's supply at a time. If the pharmacy hadn't received the Olaparib I had to wait. Usually I'd get them on time, but on the odd occasions that I didn't I'd go into fear and ring Gary's rooms or the pharmacy asking what's going on and when were my tablets going to arrive. I know I drove them a little potty when I did that because Gary very calmly but pointedly agreed with a "Yes I know" when I shared that I'd rung his office a few times because I was stressing.

So being aware of the stress and fear I was feeling around not getting my tablets on time was showing me that my peace was conditional and I wanted unconditional peace.

I realised that whilst a part of me felt the need for a safety net, life didn't always give me that option. In fact, there was many a time I'd feel confident and safe only to have that swept away. And in hind sight, not just with the cancer stuff. Living life in general, really living life, involves calculated risk, taking that chance, being willing to fail, making mistakes, losing the things we love dearly, falling over and then getting back up again. Letting go, trusting, discerning, and most importantly listening to what resonates within you. Allowing the truth of your life to unfold as it's asking to be lived.

As much as I wanted a permanent safety net, life kept showing me I wasn't going to get it.

So what do I want to do with that knowledge?

I want to find a way to really accept and live whatever life brings to me.

Knowing that life is not going to always conform to how I think things should be, I want to be able to live from a resilience within myself that knows:

Ok, this challenge/opportunity is here, how do I work with what's been given to me?

What's the best that I can do in this situation?

I want to trust my life, my process.

CHAPTER 7

Still In Remission - 2016

In 2016 I wrote a letter to each of my children telling them how honoured and grateful I was to be their mum. How they taught me the meaning of true love. They showed me so many different faces of love that I didn't know existed. They helped me to grow as a person. They taught me acceptance, tolerance and non-judgement. They helped me face some scary parent fears and they taught me to let go. At times bit by bit. Other times it felt like a band aid being ripped off as quickly as possible!! (Clearly I wasn't letting go quickly enough for them !!).

They have a natural wisdom that blows me away.

They are my greatest teachers and I love them dearly with all of my heart.

Towards the end of 2016 I was starting to feel really tired and began struggling with the quantity of Olaparib I was taking.

That was a really big year for us as my beautiful mum was quite ill and another two gorgeous grandchildren were born into our ever expanding family. So David and I were now grandparents to five children five years and under. Life was full and busy.

Mum eventually became too ill to live at home and the amount of effort it took us to get her assessed so we could get the help she needed was frustrating and hard work. I literally felt like I was banging my head on a brick wall until it was going to burst!!

(I managed to get a cold six times that year!!). There were moments when caring and lovely people would pop into Mums life, and they were a godsend, but a lot of the time it was a seemingly endless loop of doctor appointments, phone calls to organisations who rarely rang you back, hospital stays, tests, rehab then home.

Eventually mum was assessed and we were able to request a two week respite stay at a beautiful Aged Care "Resort" as we called it. She loved it there. The nurses, doctor and staff looked after her with such care and dignity. She kept asking us to extend her stay!! Which we were thankfully able to do.

Mum died on 14 September 2016. She passed peacefully and was surrounded by her family. She loved her family. We meant everything to her. I felt so blessed and privileged to have been able to sit with her in the last few days of her life.

In November of that year I also went to Byron Bay to listen to Gangaji, a Spiritual teacher I've been listening to for about ten years. I wanted to explore with her my need to never experience the terror of cancer again. I was tired of running from it. Tired of it humming in the background of my life. Tired of being scared of experiencing that feeling of terror again if cancer should come back.

My question to her was this:

How do I move out of the terror of cancer? When I'm feeling terrified I get stuck in that terror. I become that terror and I don't know how to move through it.

She offered me this:

"Can you feel the terror now?"

"No."

"What are you feeling right now?"

"Numb."

"That's ok, stay with the numbness."

I did. I couldn't move out of it.

She asked me what was happening and I told her I was still feeling numb and she said:

"That's ok, I'm not asking you to do anything with the numbness. Not asking you to get rid of it or anything."

And for some reason, I feel because she was so accepting of where I was at and not judging it as wrong, I suddenly felt this beautiful peace rise up in me.

Gangaji asked me if I'd asked this peace to come.

I hadn't. I just felt it spontaneously flow up and through me. And I could see how the numbness I'd previously felt was protecting me from feeling the terror and how I was judging that as wrong. Feeling and hearing Gangaji accept my numbness helped me to realise it was ok. I'd been holding a belief that said I shouldn't feel fear, terror or numbness. By allowing it to be ok I felt released from that belief. She helped me to feel more compassion for myself. To allow fear to be present and feel compassion for that part of me that was so scared. I was so grateful for that experience.

Towards the end of this year I decided to cut back my dosage of Olaparib to see if my energy levels would improve. They did for a while but by 2017 I was struggling again so I reduced them further.

CHAPTER 8

Exhaustion - 2017

So now I'm on half the dosage I'd started in 2015. My tumour markers are still stable and I'm feeling ok. Still tired, but not too bad.

Family life is busy. It's early 2017. We're expecting our sixth grandchild in August, and David's dad isn't well.

During this time I'd had a scare that the cancer might be back. I kept getting this weird pain/sensation under my left breast just over the top of my ribs that reminded me of the pain I felt when I was first diagnosed in 2011. The pain started on a Friday night. Initially I felt disappointed, sad, and scared. I thought I had come to a more peaceful place about this cancer, but the strong fear I felt was showing me I hadn't. David took me out over that weekend and I remember us walking along a beautiful beach near Sorrento. Usually sitting by the ocean and listening to the waves calms me and I can connect to the surrounding beauty, but I noticed that this time I wasn't feeling anything. I felt totally numb and couldn't connect to anyone or anything. I went to my GP the following Monday and he sent me for a CT scan. It was clear.

I also requested a mental health plan to see a psychologist. I wanted to get over this fear once and for all. I was so tired of it popping up whenever I felt tired or unwell. I hated how it crept into my life and disrupted my happiness and peace. I just wanted to be free of this fear - permanently.

I decided to find a psychologist that was closer to home. And I found beautiful Vicki.

On my first visit I remember saying to her:

"This is what I want.

I want to be at peace with this cancer.

I want to feel ok whether cancer is in my life or not. I'm over being scared of it.

I want help in finding permanent peace."

To which Vicki replied,

"Wow big ask."

She helped me to understand and live, that fear is a part of life. That it's ok to feel it. She asked me what I'd do if a child or someone I loved came to me, scared and worried. I told her I'd hug them and reassure them that they're not alone, that I loved them dearly and was there for them no matter what. To which Vicki asked me: "Can you do that for yourself in your moments of fear with cancer?"

My answer was a definite yes.

I've been practicing what Vicki was asking for years, but because my fear of cancer was so strong I'd freeze whenever cancer was the issue. Fear of mostly everything else in my life- yes - compassion would arise and my self talk was gentle and kind. If the fear was around cancer, all I wanted to do was be free of it. Vicki helped me to offer that same compassion, gentleness and kindness to my fear of cancer. I still offer myself that love and kindness to this day whenever that fear arises. And when I catch my self judgement around that fear still being there, I take a deep breath and give myself a loving break.

I saw Gary a few weeks after the scan and he told me my markers were good.

I decided to start having acupuncture to see if it would help revive my energy levels.

I always left those sessions feeling great, but it didn't last. By the time our grandson was born in August I was exhausted.

My next visit to Gary showed me why. My tumour markers had jumped from a steady 12 to 29. I looked at him and said:

"It's back then."

To which Gary replied:

"Not necessarily. We'll wait six weeks and see what happens."

But I knew it was back. I said to Gary that my history has always shown that as soon as my markers move - It's back.

He tried to reassure me by saying: "Let's wait and see. Have another blood test in six weeks and we'll make a decision from there.

Try not to worry."

I looked over the top of my glasses at him and said:

"That's not in my personality Gary." He just smiled and agreed.

This time though I felt no fear.

I felt heavy. I didn't cry. None of the usual emotions I'd felt in the past came up. I just felt this heavy acceptance.

Six weeks later my markers are higher again, well over the 30 mark which indicates cancer is present so I'm off for a PET and a CT scan which shows a small lump behind my bladder but no obvious cancer anywhere else. I go to see Tom, the surgeon I had in 2011, to have the lump removed and to have a laparoscopy to make sure there's no cancer anywhere else.

David and I are pretty excited at the prospect of there being only one lump and that it's removable because in our minds that's so different to how the cancer has presented in the past. Usually I get a lot of tiny tumours that can only be treated with chemo.

12 October 2017 I'm in the Epworth Hospital in Melbourne waiting to have my procedure done. My prep nurse is lovely. She's also had a brush with breast cancer. So many people seem to get it now. Or am I just more aware of it because of my personal circumstances? I'm feeling a bit nervous but I'm also ok because I love going under anesthetic. It's such a lovely deep and relaxing sleep!!!!

Tom visits me the day after my surgery and tells me the lump isn't cancer, but unfortunately there is cancer present over my stomach area. Ironic, but I'm not surprised, and I feel disappointed - but only slightly this time.

I go back and see Gary and we organise my chemo treatments.

I remember David and I having a bet as to how high my markers would be. The winner got dinner. I won. I thought afterwards: "I didn't think that one through very well. I should have asked for diamonds!!"

So my regime of chemo started again in October.

There was a chemo I'd had a few years ago that I didn't cope with very well so I asked Gary not to give me that one again.

Physically I didn't recover as well as I had in the past. Emotionally though I wasn't in the terror I thought I might feel with cancer returning. I still had my moments, but they weren't as overwhelming as they used to be. Spiritually I felt really happy. I felt love. I felt the beauty of life and I felt compassion for what my body was going through.

I was pretty tired over Christmas and felt some grief around not having the energy I would have liked to have had with our family, but then I was also learning to live within my body's capabilities. Something I never did when I was younger. I used to push my body even when it was screaming at me that it was tired. I'd just keep going. Eventually I had to listen. I didn't want, nor did I have, the energy to keep pushing myself physically. I wanted to be kinder to myself in all areas of my life.

That wanting later showed me how I was still subtly pushing myself and compromising my wellbeing.

CHAPTER 9

Remission - 2018

In February 2018 I'm thankfully in remission again. Physically exhausted, emotionally ok and spiritually great.

Gary put me on a drug called Avastin, which I was receiving during my chemo treatments and will continue to receive on a three-weekly basis until December 2018/January 2019. It prevents new blood vessels from forming which starves the cancer as it's got nothing to feed on. I also resumed Lynparza (Olaparib) in March of this year.

In late June I asked Gary if I could have Avastin every four weeks instead of every three. I was starting to feel tired again. He said yes, but that there was no evidence that it would be as effective. I went straight into fear, told Gary as much, and he suggested I go home and think about what I'd like to do.

I went downstairs to Day Oncology for my Avastin infusion with a couple of uncomfortable emotions running in me. My first was disappointment when I noticed how quickly fear popped up again, the second was doubt. Am I doing the best thing for my body if I go from three weeks to four on the Avastin? I didn't know what to do. Fear and doubt were simultaneously present. I decided to ask one of the oncology nurses that has been on this journey with me since 2011 to be my sounding board. I trust and value her wisdom and compassion.

So while I was receiving my infusion I asked Jo her thoughts on what I was thinking. She said because she's not an oncologist she couldn't advise me medically and that her advice would be to trust and be guided by what Gary recommended. But as he was ok with me having Avastin every four weeks I still felt confused. This is what Jo kindly offered me:

She reminded me of my tendency to fall into regret. I had regretted dropping my dosage of Lynparza. Cancer may have returned regardless of the amount I was taking, there's no absolute knowing whether that's true or not. But mentally and emotionally I regretted that choice.

How would I feel if I changed my infusions from every 3 weeks to every 4 and the cancer came back? Would I step into regret? I knew instantly that I would. I still wanted to live as long as I could being cancer free.

Jo also offered me this:

"Sylv, I don't know many people that are going through what you're going through who look after as many people as you do. You need to learn to say that little word NO more often."

I burst into tears and realised I was doing with the Avastin what I'd done with the Lynparza. Reduce the dose so I would have the energy to be able to do more. I was still missing the energetic me I used to be. And I didn't like not being able to push through my tiredness.

Thanks Jo. Another beautiful teacher and light in my life.

I can't and don't want to do that to myself anymore.

So on my next visit to Gary my decision was easy. No fear, no doubt.

Avastin every three weeks please.

CHAPTER 10

Realisations And How I Feel Today As I Write This Chapter – October 2018

Realising I could want with all of my heart to live cancer free and to accept that that may not be what unfolds has been very freeing for me.

I can still love, still live, laugh, and embrace all that life brings to me. That cancer isn't a death sentence to the whole of my being. That life is still lived and loved regardless of whether cancer is here or not.

That just because my physical survival wants to live forever doesn't mean it will. In fact it can't.

Even those beautiful miraculous people that have had spontaneous remissions from cancer will physically die one day.

It doesn't matter what we die from ultimately. It matters what we're living for. What we've chosen to dedicate our lives to. How kind we're choosing to be to ourselves and others. Our planet. What choices am I making while living in this amazing body that's given so much. Been through soooo much, yet keeps on healing and going?

Yes, cancer kept returning. And some people who hold the belief that our minds and thoughts have the power to influence all outcomes in our lives, might say my thought process kept bringing it back. The fears I felt gave cancer power. Maybe they did, maybe they didn't. I don't know the absolute truth behind the reasons.

Inheriting the BRCA 1 Gene mutation may have had some relevance, but then for some reason people with that genetic history may never get cancer. My dad is 84, is a carrier of the mutation, is the biggest worry wart I've ever known and has never had cancer in his life.

The truth for me now is it doesn't matter why it kept coming back. I choose to focus on how I can live my life now. How can I honour the life I've been blessed with now. How can I best serve what life brings me? That's my focus these days.

It feels too restrictive, too contracting for me to constantly scan and look for the reasons behind cancer returning.

I still choose to eat organic and healthy most of the time, this time though it's because I care about myself. I exercise, I have regular energy healings and kinesiology. I visit my GP if my body is feeling out of sync physically, I can you tube and read books written by the spiritual teachers I love and attend silent retreats with them via the internet.

I have my psychologist, family and friends for my emotional wellbeing and my oncologist and caring nurses for regular drug administration and blood tests.

I have me. My resilience, my self compassion and love, my unfolding life to be lived.

I don't know how I'll be if cancer returns. My feeling is I'll get on with what needs to be done in a loving, honest and informed way.

Fear might pop up and if it does I'll acknowledge it and soothe that part of me that's fearful, all the time knowing that the part of me that's seeing the fear, seeing the comforting, is where I'm choosing to live from.

And from that living, no safety net is needed

CHAPTER 11

Gratitude

My Beloved Husband David:

Thank you for sharing this dance of life with me. Your love, support and honesty have been amazing. You never backed away from the heartache of this journey. You stayed calm when I spun out emotionally and stepped in and made the calls that needed to be made so that we were making informed decisions from facts not the stories and fears in my mind. You stand beside me no matter what.

I love you with all of my heart

My Beautiful Children :

To Chris who was an absolute rock of optimism googling and reading up on all the therapies that were available to me.

To Di whose strong belief that I'll be ok and at peace when my death is here.

And to Brendon for bringing peace back into my heart.

Thank you thank you thank you.

These are some of the beautiful wisdoms you shared with me:

CHRIS:

"There's new treatments coming out all the time mum"

Thank you to my amazing oldest son who was my rock when I needed to talk through my emotional fears about cancer. You never backed away from me when I was really scared and downhearted. You always looked at the positives.

A lot of the original questions for Gary when I was first diagnosed came from you hon. I'm so grateful to you for your tireless searching on the internet for trials and new research that was coming out.

And for your clarity. When I was lost in my emotional pit of "what if's" and regrets, you stayed calm and helped me to see it all from a different perspective.

I love you with all of my heart.

DIANE:

"Embrace the germs!
(My wisdom for your OCD problems!!)"

OMG Di, I couldn't stop laughing when I read that in the beautiful diary you gave me.

"To write down all the positive, good things in your life mum"

Thank you my gorgeous daughter for your humour and love. I love what you wrote in my diary!! For your strong belief in my being able to be at peace when it comes time for me to die. For the beautiful text you sent me telling me you'd all be by my side always and reassuring me that I'd be ok.

I love you with all of my heart.

<u>BRENDON:</u>

**"There's something there and it's ok not to know what it is.
And it's peaceful and it's loving.
It's so natural.
It's like being born back into where you first came from."**

Thank you to my beautiful youngest son who shared this heart felt wisdom with me in 2011. When I told you I was terrified of dying because I really didn't know what happens when we die, you offered this beautiful insight to me. I could feel the genuine peace you were coming from and that peace transferred to me. It stopped the shaking in my body. I'll always be grateful that I can share my thoughts about death with you so openly and honestly hon.

I love you with all of my heart.

My Grandchildren Indi, Harper, Addi, Evie, Jimmy, Wilder and Reef:

To my adorable, heart opening grandchildren. You fill me with so much love, joy and happiness. You're the sunshine in my life.

I love you all so very, very much.

My Children's Partners Sarah, Beecher and Jess:

Thank you for your understanding and caring and for being such awesome parents!! You're raising caring, resilient children. The world is so blessed!!

I love you all very much.

My Family and Friends:

Where would I be without my family and friends!! Thank you for your shared laughter, great lunches and dinners. Deep and meaningful conversations, prayers, honesty and love. You make my life sooooooo much richer!!

I love you all very, very much.

CHAPTER 12

Professor Gary Richardson AM - Oncologist

Questions

Q. Why did you choose to become an Oncologist?

The variety, the technology, and the patient contact. Plus, great mentors.

Q. When you're seeing a patient for the first time what's going through your mind?

Ensure I have all the information so I can make the best decision for each patient.

Q. What are your hopes and goals for your patients?

To help them as much as possible. This may mean cure, prolonging life, or just relieving symptoms.

Q. So many people have such strong fears around this disease. It seems to be so terrifying for most of us. Do we need to be so afraid of cancer?

My motto is to only worry about the things you can change. With cancer, a lot is very treatable, but despite this people have great fear of the disease. Much like fear of sharks, it is overestimated.

Q. What are your thoughts about death?

Inevitable.

Q. What's your philosophy for living?

Never let a chance go by and always do your best.

My own personal experience of you Gary is this:

When I'm sitting in your office, I get a sense that you see cancer as a challenging disease, *that in most cases, if it's not curable, it's definitely manageable, and not something that we necessarily need to be so afraid of.

You're compassionate when fear's present and at times more serious when the news isn't great, but you always have an air of positivity, confidence, and an awesome sense of humour.   Thanks for being who you are.

* **NB:** In the above paragraph where I've written "that in most cases, if it it's not curable, it's definitely manageable" - Gary has corrected me (regarding the "in most cases" comment). His correction is: "Not true, 70% now curable"

My feeling when I read this was - YAY!! That's awesome.

CHAPTER 13

Searching for Peace

By: Sylvia Fortnam

When I was given the diagnosis of ovarian cancer in 2011, I started looking for a miracle cure and emotional peace around my own death. On reflection I feel that the miracle cure was my way of finding peace around dying because if I was cured, death has been delayed. I've been given more time and I don't have to think about death anymore.

It felt like: Miracle Cure = No Death = Peace.   Brilliant!! Problem solved.

In 2013 ovarian cancer returned with the diagnosis that it would keep returning. And so my search for peace around death became even more urgent, as it really hit home that dying one day was a given. No escaping it – no avoiding it.

In 2011 I expanded my reading on people who had been miraculously cured. (I've been interested in reading/learning complementary therapies since 1999). Spontaneous remissions/healings, eating only raw foods, meditation, visualisation, holy healing waters, vitamin C infusions, spiritual healings and more. I understood that the reason for this was the hope that I may be cured as well if I followed the same regimes. And whilst I do believe such healings are true for some people, for most of us that are diagnosed with an ongoing illness – spontaneous remission doesn't occur.

Some might suggest that any cancer patient who hasn't been cured wasn't mentally positive enough or they didn't eat enough organic foods/juices or take the right vitamins/herbs, visualise or meditate properly. Some might suggest it's Karma. And please don't think I'm against any of the above therapies, I'm not. I've tried a few of them myself (and still receive treatment for and practice some), and I've found them to be very loving, nurturing and life enhancing experiences for me. But did it stop my particular cancer from returning? No. (So far cancer's been in my life 4 times). Did it stop me fearing death? No. I was terrified when I was first diagnosed with Stage 3c ovarian cancer 4 years ago, and then tested positive to the BRCA 1 mutation in 2012. I still step into fear every now and then.

I've had the odd therapist and well-meaning friends suggest that the reason this cancer kept returning was because I still held some fear around it. I'd been asked how I was going to think differently to stop this cancer coming back. And for a while I felt cancer was my fault, that I was doing something wrong because I couldn't cure it. I blamed myself. I could see that they were making these suggestions because they genuinely cared and believed in what they were saying. And they wanted me to be well.

I did try to find a way of not being afraid of cancer and death, but what I discovered instead was, that for me, fear is a part of being human and that to acknowledge fear is present is ok. Does it overwhelm me? It used to. I used to *become* the fear and terror. Most days now if fear arises it arises in the space of love and acceptance. Fear is here, sometimes sadness is here, sometimes extreme tiredness is present, mostly love and laughter with my husband, children, grandchildren and extended family and friends is here.

When overwhelming emotion is present and I can't see my way through it, I ask for help.

And I'm ok with all of this at the moment.

The stark reality I've come to is: OMG this body isn't going to last forever!!"

Illness has forced me to look at my mortality. And I've come to the conclusion that the majority of us don't spontaneously heal.

My search for peace has led me to ask myself:
"Since death is inevitable, (eventually even those who have been miraculously cured will also die), *How Do I Want To Live?"*

My husband David and I were talking the other night about what would be the best way to find inner peace with a diagnosis of cancer re-occurring, which for me reminds me of my mortality, and usually triggers some kind of emotion. My thoughts were that if we were able to speak more openly about death it wouldn't be such a scary thing. That maybe, through being enriched and inspired by someone's living *and* dying, there could be peace in accepting that death is a given instead of chasing the hope that "I'll be miraculously cured of this disease", because to me, I might be cured of this disease or I might not.

I'm not saying fear of death is bad or wrong. To me it's natural. We want to survive. But the true and honest fact is that we will all die one day. Death is a part of living on this planet, it's part of Life's Cycle. And yes, I get scared sometimes when I look at my own death. And sometimes I feel really peaceful because I know I can't stop death from happening and there's a letting go of hanging on so tightly. I literally breathe out and relax – sometimes.

What David shared with me felt so beautiful. What if we just accepted that everyone copes with a life-threatening diagnosis in their own way? Some people decide, "Right then, I'm living what's left of my life eating, drinking and doing what I want." Some people can't stop crying, some are terrified, some decide to fight it tooth and nail and some quietly accept it.

Wow! When I heard these words something inside me softened. How loving is that!!

To accept that we all have our own unique way of coping with life's challenges. There's freedom in that. And for me, a peacefulness in that acceptance.

I still want to do the best I can to live a long and happy life, and I know that even doing this and having the best medical, complementary and spiritual team in the world will not stop this body from dying one day. So what to do?

Knowing, as a fact, that this body will die and there's nothing I can do to stop that from happening:

How do I want to live now? In this moment?

My answer is this:

For me, in this moment, I want to live authentically.

I want to live my life from my heart, following what enlivens me with compassion, kindness and courage.

I want my beautiful family, friends, medical, complementary and spiritual team to know how much I cherish and love them; and

I want to feel deeply the gratitude I have for the life I've been blessed with so far.

My reason for writing this article is not to take away anyone's hope of a cure, nor to increase any fears about death. It's my hope that no-one blames themselves if a cure doesn't occur. That their life isn't lived in regret or blame if the diagnosis isn't what they were hoping for. That in accepting that there's nothing we can do to prevent death occurring one day, we embrace life with more love and self-acceptance and hopefully find peace, however that unfolds for us. To do the best we can with what we've got and where we're at in any given moment. To reach out for help when we need it. And to be gentle with ourselves.

To me, cancer isn't a fight. I personally find that concept exhausting. To me, cancer is a journey. It's still a part of living. It's changed how I live. It's challenged and brought change to a lot of my personal and spiritual beliefs. I feel it's deepened my wanting to be more loving, honest and sincere with myself and in my connections with people and life.

And with the help of my beautiful oncology psychologist Jane, it's still teaching me (and constantly reminding me), to live fully and from this moment.

With much love to you all wherever you are on your own personal journeys.

Sylv xx

Written: 2015, Revised: October 2018

About the Author

After graduating in the Carl Rogers method of counselling, Sylvia practiced as a counsellor for a number of years, always working towards helping her clients find their own sense of self-empowerment, self-love and self-trust.

She also loved offering Indian Head Massage to clients who wanted a break from their mind and some relief from the stresses of their everyday life.

Having studied Kinesiology and qualifying as a Level One Kinesiologist Sylvia incorporated this learning in both her counselling and massage sessions.

She has a love for spiritual growth and was involved in a caring and compassionate Tibetan Buddhist Community with spiritual teacher Lama Tendar for three years where she learned the philosophy of Tibetan Buddhism and attended various courses and Empowerments.

She continues to connect to the spiritual teachers she resonates with via the internet and, whenever possible, in person.

Sylvia is the mother of three adult children and grandmother to seven grandchildren. She lives near the beautiful Mornington Peninsula in Victoria, Australia with her husband of 42 years and their bouncy miniature bullterrier Lucy.

www.ingramcontent.com/pod-product-compliance
Lightning Source LLC
LaVergne TN
LVHW021548080426
835509LV00019B/2898